Rice Diet

A Review, Analysis, and Beginner's Step by Step Overview

copyright © 2019 Bruce Ackerberg

All rights reserved No part of this book may be reproduced, or stored in a retrieval system, or transmitted in any form or by any means, electronic, mechanical, photocopying, recording, or otherwise, without express written permission of the publisher.

Disclaimer

By reading this disclaimer, you are accepting the terms of the disclaimer in full. If you disagree with this disclaimer, please do not read the guide.

All of the content within this guide is provided for informational and educational purposes only, and should not be accepted as independent medical or other professional advice. The author is not a doctor, physician, nurse, mental health provider, or registered nutritionist/dietician. Therefore, using and reading this guide does not establish any form of a physician-patient relationship.

Always consult with a physician or another qualified health provider with any issues or questions you might have regarding any sort of medical condition. Do not ever disregard any qualified professional medical advice or delay seeking that advice because of anything you have read in this guide. The information in this guide is not intended to be any sort of medical advice and should not be used in lieu of any medical advice by a licensed and qualified medical professional.

The information in this guide has been compiled from a variety of known sources. However, the author cannot attest to or guarantee the accuracy of each source and thus should not be held liable for any errors or omissions.

You acknowledge that the publisher of this guide will not be held liable for any loss or damage of any kind incurred as a result of this guide or the reliance on any information provided within this guide. You acknowledge and agree that you assume all risk and responsibility for any action you undertake in response to the information in this guide.

Using this guide does not guarantee any particular result (e.g., weight loss or a cure). By reading this guide, you acknowledge that there are no guarantees to any specific outcome or results you can expect.

All product names, diet plans, or names used in this guide are for identification purposes only and are the property of their respective owners. The use of these names does not imply endorsement. All other trademarks cited herein are the property of their respective owners.

Where applicable, this guide is not intended to be a substitute for the original work of this diet plan and is, at most, a supplement to the original work for this diet plan and never a direct substitute. This guide is a personal expression of the facts of that diet plan.

Where applicable, persons shown in the cover images are stock photography models and the publisher has obtained the rights to use the images through license agreements with third-party stock image companies.

Table of Contents

Introduction	7
What Is a Chronic Disease?	10
Causes of Chronic Disease	11
Symptoms of Chronic Disease	14
Diagnosis and Medical Treatments for Chronic Disease	19
Diagnosis of chronic disease	19
Medical treatments for chronic disease	21
Lifestyle changes for chronic diseases	24
What Is a Rice Diet?	29
Scientific Evidence Supporting the Rice Diet	30
Modern Interpretations and Future Research	33
Principles of the Rice Diet	34
Benefits of the Rice Diet	38
Disadvantages of the Rice Diet	43
Common Challenges and Solutions	46
Final Tips for Long-Term Success	51
The 5-Step Guide to Getting Started on the Rice Diet	53
Step 1: Consult with a healthcare professional	53
Step 2: Stock Up on the Essentials	54
Step 3: Establish Your Meal Plan	55
Step 4: Gradually Introduce Rice	56
Step 5: Keep track and adjust as needed	57
The Three Phases of the Rice Diet	59
Phase 1 of the Rice Diet: Your Comprehensive Guide	59
Phase 2 of the Rice Diet: Understanding the Process	62
Phase 3 of the Rice Diet: Lifestyle Change and Maintenance	64
Foods to Eat in the Rice Diet	68
Foods to Avoid in the Rice Diet	72
Adjusting the Rice Diet for Specific Needs	76

Adjusting the Rice Diet for Diabetes	76
Adjusting the Rice Diet for Hypertension	77
Adjusting the Rice Diet for Gluten Intolerance	79
General Considerations for Tailoring the Diet	80
Success Stories and Testimonials	**82**
Sample Menus	**84**
Lacto-Vegetarian Diet	84
Vegetarian Plus	85
Sample Recipes	**87**
Low-Calorie French Toast	88
Bread Stew	89
Garbanzo Stew	91
Tilapia Jasmine Rice	93
Yellow Rice	95
Cauliflower Rice Substitute	96
Conclusion	**98**
FAQs	**100**
References and Helpful Links	**103**

Introduction

Chronic diseases are on the rise in the modern world and have become a significant cause for concern for healthcare systems worldwide. According to the World Health Organization (WHO), chronic diseases such as diabetes, stroke, heart disease, and cancer are responsible for 70% of deaths worldwide. Therefore, it is crucial to find ways to prevent and manage these debilitating conditions effectively.

One such approach is the Rice Diet. The Rice Diet was created in the early 1930s by Dr. Walter Kempner at Duke University in North Carolina, USA. Originally, it was designed to treat hypertension (high blood pressure), but it has since become a popular choice for managing and preventing chronic diseases.

The Rice Diet is a low-fat, low-sodium, and low-protein diet that is primarily based on rice, fruits, and vegetables. It limits the intake of animal products, processed foods, and added sugars. Instead, it encourages the consumption of whole foods, such as whole grains, fruits, and vegetables, which are nutrient-dense and high in fiber.

The Rice Diet is effective in managing and preventing chronic diseases such as hypertension, diabetes, cardiovascular disease, and kidney disease. A study published in The Journal of Nutrition in 2002 showed that the Rice Diet improved blood pressure, blood sugar levels, and cholesterol profiles in hypertensive and diabetic patients.

The benefits of the Rice Diet are not restricted to physical health alone. Research has also shown that the Rice Diet has positive effects on mental health. A study conducted in 2019 found that the Rice Diet improved depression, anxiety, and stress levels among participants.

In this guide, we will talk about the following:

- What is a chronic disease?
- Symptoms of Chronic Disease
- Causes of chronic disease
- Lifestyle Changes for Chronic Disease
- Medical Treatments for Chronic Diseases
- What is the rice diet good for?
- Principles of the Rice Diet
- Benefits and Disadvantages of the Rice Diet
- The Three Phases of the Rice Diet
- Foods to Eat and Avoid in the Rice Diet
- A 5-Step Guide to Getting Started on the Rice Diet

Whether you're dealing with diabetes, heart disease, obesity, or another chronic disease, the Rice Diet can be a powerful tool for improving your health and quality of life. By following the principles of the Rice Diet and making sustainable lifestyle changes, you can reduce your risk of complications and feel your best.

What Is a Chronic Disease?

Chronic diseases are long-term illnesses that affect millions of people worldwide. Chronic diseases can last for many years, often for the person's entire lifetime, and can interfere with daily life activities. Examples of chronic diseases include heart disease, diabetes, stroke, cancer, and respiratory diseases.

Unlike acute diseases, which have a sudden onset and are usually resolved quickly, chronic diseases develop slowly over time and often have no known cure. They can be caused by various factors, including genetics, lifestyle factors such as poor nutrition and a lack of exercise, and exposure to environmental factors such as air pollution.

Chronic diseases can significantly impact a person's quality of life and require ongoing medical attention, treatment, and management. They are responsible for a significant burden on healthcare systems worldwide, accounting for a high percentage of healthcare costs.

Causes of Chronic Disease

The causes of chronic diseases are complex and varied, but some of the most common risk factors include:

1. **Genetics**

    Research suggests that genetics plays a crucial role in the development of chronic diseases, including cardiovascular disease and cancer. Individuals may inherit genetic mutations that increase their susceptibility to these illnesses.

    Such mutations may affect the functioning of genes responsible for regulating key processes in the body, such as cell growth and repair, immune response, and metabolism. While genetic predisposition does not necessarily guarantee the onset of disease, it certainly increases the likelihood of developing it.

2. **Lifestyle Factors**

    Poor nutrition, a lack of physical activity, and exposure to environmental toxins are known to be major causes of chronic diseases. When individuals lead an unhealthy lifestyle that involves these factors, it can create an environment in the body that promotes inflammation, which is a risk factor for diseases such as diabetes and heart disease.

To reduce the risk of chronic disease development, individuals need to adopt a healthy lifestyle that includes a balanced diet, regular exercise, and avoidance of environmental toxins.

3. Infections

Viral or bacterial infections are known to be a significant contributor to certain chronic illnesses like hepatitis, HIV/AIDS, and tuberculosis. These infections may cause long-term complications even after the infection has been treated.

According to medical experts, chronic viral infections can lead to chronic inflammation, which may result in irreversible damage to vital organs such as the liver, causing liver cancer or cirrhosis. Similarly, untreated HIV infection may lead to the development of acquired immune deficiency syndrome (AIDS), which adversely affects the immune system and may cause other infections or cancers.

4. Age

A major contributor to the development of chronic diseases among older individuals is the natural process of aging. Over time, the body undergoes wear and tear that affects various parts, including the immune system.

As a result, elderly people are more prone to infections and chronic illnesses. Other factors that increase the risk of chronic diseases in old age are poor nutrition and a sedentary lifestyle. People who fail to maintain a healthy diet and regular exercise routine are more likely to develop conditions such as type 2 diabetes, heart disease, and high blood pressure.

5. **Psychological Factors**

Chronic stress and depression can cause significant harm to an individual's overall health, increasing the risk of developing chronic diseases such as heart disease and stroke. The negative effects of these psychological factors can stem from unhealthy coping mechanisms such as overeating and smoking, which can further exacerbate the risk of chronic diseases.

Overeating can lead to weight gain and obesity, while smoking can increase the risk of lung cancer and heart disease.

To avoid these complications, individuals need to manage their stress levels and seek help if necessary to improve mental health. Additionally, regular exercise, a balanced diet, and adequate rest are important for promoting overall health and reducing the risk of chronic diseases. Adopting a healthy lifestyle is key to preventing or managing chronic illnesses.

Symptoms of Chronic Disease

The symptoms of chronic diseases vary greatly depending on the condition and its severity. In general, however, a few common symptoms that are associated with many chronic diseases include:

1. **Fatigue**

    Chronic fatigue is a commonly reported symptom among people with chronic diseases. This persistent sense of exhaustion can be attributed to a variety of factors, including inflammation and poor nutrition.

    These underlying conditions can cause fatigue by interfering with the body's ability to absorb necessary nutrients, leading to a lack of energy. Additionally, inflammation can cause significant discomfort and contribute to feelings of tiredness. Individuals experiencing chronic fatigue may benefit from seeking medical attention to address the underlying causes of this symptom.

2. **Pain**

    Chronic pain is a significant symptom among individuals suffering from chronic diseases, such as arthritis, fibromyalgia, and multiple sclerosis. Patients often struggle to manage their chronic pain, which can negatively impact their physical, emotional, and cognitive well-being.

3. **Difficulty breathing**

   People suffering from chronic respiratory diseases such as asthma and chronic obstructive pulmonary disease (COPD) commonly experience difficulty breathing or shortness of breath. These symptoms may be triggered by physical activity, environmental factors such as pollution, or respiratory infections.

   Chronic inflammation and damage to the airways leading to obstruction and reduced lung function are hallmark features of these conditions. Furthermore, consistent and effective management of these symptoms is crucial for managing the overall health and quality of life of individuals with respiratory diseases.

4. **Cognitive Issues**

   Cognitive impairments are common symptoms of chronic diseases like Alzheimer's and Parkinson's disease. These conditions can cause difficulties in memory, thinking, and decision-making. People with Alzheimer's may struggle to remember important details or past events, while those with Parkinson's may experience a slowing down of their mental processes.

5. **Digestive Problems**

   Chronic diseases like IBS and Crohn's disease can lead to troublesome digestive symptoms. These conditions mainly cause distressing symptoms such as diarrhea, constipation, and stomach pain. IBS is a common condition that can cause abdominal discomfort and altered bowel habits.

   On the other hand, Crohn's disease is a chronic inflammatory bowel disease that can affect the digestive tract from the mouth to the anus. Treatment for these chronic diseases involves managing symptoms and may require medication, dietary changes, or lifestyle modifications to provide relief.

6. **Skin Issues**

   Psoriasis and eczema are two chronic skin diseases that can cause a range of symptoms, including rashes, redness, and persistent itching. These conditions occur due to immune system response, leading to inflammation and thickened skin.

   Psoriasis is characterized by patches of scaly, silvery skin that can be painful and itchy, while eczema is a more generalized rash that can appear anywhere on the body. Both conditions are not contagious and can be managed with medical treatment and lifestyle changes. It is essential to seek medical advice if one experiences these symptoms to prevent further complications.

7. **Mood Disorders**

   Chronic diseases are known to be associated with mood disorders such as depression and anxiety as they can negatively impact an individual's overall physical and mental well-being. Studies have shown a direct link between chronic diseases, their symptoms, and the development of mood disorders.

   For instance, people with chronic pain are more likely to develop depression and anxiety as their symptoms can be debilitating and limit their daily activities. Similarly, individuals with chronic illnesses such as diabetes and heart disease are also at a higher risk of developing mood disorders due to the physical strain and emotional burden of the disease.

8. **Frequent Infections**

   Chronic diseases can lead to a weakened immune system, increasing the likelihood of frequent infections such as urinary tract infections (UTIs) or pneumonia. This is due to the disease-causing ongoing inflammation in the body, which over time can damage the immune system.

Additionally, certain medications used to manage chronic diseases can also suppress the immune system, further increasing the risk of infections.

It is important to note that each chronic disease can cause different symptoms, and symptoms may vary in severity from person to person. Symptoms may also change over time as the disease progresses. Individuals with chronic diseases need to work closely with their healthcare providers to manage symptoms and improve their overall health.

Diagnosis and Medical Treatments for Chronic Disease

Now that we have discussed the potential impact of chronic diseases on mental health, it is essential to understand how these conditions are diagnosed and treated.

Diagnosis of chronic disease

Chronic diseases are typically long-lasting conditions that can negatively impact an individual's physical and mental health. Some of the most common chronic diseases include heart disease, diabetes, arthritis, and cancer.

Here are some of the methods that doctors typically use to diagnose chronic diseases:

1. *Medical History:* A doctor will begin by asking about an individual's medical history, including any underlying health conditions, medications they're currently taking, and any relevant family medical history.
2. *Physical Examination:* Doctors will perform a physical examination to look for signs of chronic

diseases such as high blood pressure, abnormal heart rhythm, or a mass or lump that could indicate cancer.
3. *Lab Tests:* Lab tests can also be used to diagnose chronic diseases. For example, doctors can measure blood glucose levels to diagnose diabetes, or they may look for elevated levels of cholesterol or other blood lipids to diagnose heart disease.
4. *Imaging Tests:* Imaging tests such as X-rays, CT scans, and MRIs can help doctors diagnose chronic diseases affecting the bones, muscles, and organs.
5. *Genetic Testing:* In some cases, genetic testing can help doctors diagnose chronic diseases that run in families, such as cystic fibrosis or sickle cell anemia.
6. *Biopsy:* A biopsy involves removing a small sample of tissue from the body and examining it under a microscope. Biopsies can help diagnose cancer and other chronic diseases.

Diagnosing chronic diseases can be complex, and doctors may use a combination of these methods to arrive at an accurate diagnosis. Early diagnosis is crucial for treating chronic diseases and minimizing the risk of serious complications, so it's important to seek medical attention if you are experiencing symptoms or have a family history of chronic diseases.

Medical treatments for chronic disease

When it comes to treating chronic diseases, there are a variety of medical treatments available. Depending on the type and severity of the disease, some treatments may be more effective than others.

1. **Medications**

    Doctors prescribe medications to manage symptoms and minimize the progression of chronic diseases. These treatments typically target specific conditions and can vary depending on the individual's needs. For instance, high blood pressure patients may receive drugs that decrease their blood pressure levels, whilst those with diabetes may require insulin to regulate glucose in their blood.

    To optimize effectiveness, medications should be taken under medical supervision and coupled with healthy lifestyle habits such as exercise, a well-balanced diet, and stress management techniques.

2. **Surgery**

    Surgery can be an effective treatment for chronic diseases such as severe osteoarthritis and heart disease. Joint replacement surgery is recommended for individuals with damaged and worn-out joints due to osteoarthritis.

Meanwhile, people with heart disease may require bypass surgery to reroute blood flow around blocked arteries. These surgeries can provide relief from chronic pain and improve the overall quality of life for individuals living with chronic diseases. Despite the benefits, surgery is often considered a last resort after other treatments have failed and may come with risks and complications.

3. **Physical therapy**

Physical therapy is an important treatment method for chronic conditions that impair mobility or cause persistent pain. Approved regimens may involve diverse techniques such as targeted exercises, stretches, and specialized equipment to mitigate symptoms and improve overall function.

This medical intervention has been established as an effective long-term option for managing chronic ailments, with a growing body of evidence supporting its efficacy in mitigating pain, improving range of motion, and enhancing strength and flexibility.

4. **Occupational therapy**

Occupational therapy is a critical medical treatment for patients with chronic diseases, helping them to perform daily activities and maintain their independence. It offers a range of techniques that aid in pain management, including modifications to the home or workplace and the use of adaptive equipment.

Occupational therapy also provides support by helping patients with long-term conditions develop skills and strategies to manage their symptoms, leading to increased satisfaction and improved quality of life. By enhancing patients' ability to participate in daily activities, occupational therapy plays a crucial role in managing chronic diseases.

5. **Lifestyle changes**

    Even with medical treatments, making certain lifestyle changes can help manage chronic diseases. Quitting smoking, for example, can reduce the risk of heart disease and cancer. Eating a healthy diet can improve blood sugar control, cholesterol levels, and blood pressure.

    Regular exercise can improve overall health, help manage weight, and reduce the risk of chronic diseases, such as diabetes and heart disease. These lifestyle changes can also help manage symptoms and potentially reduce the need for medication in some cases.

These treatments can help manage symptoms and improve quality of life, but it is important to remember that many chronic diseases have no cure. Treatment plans should be tailored to each individual's specific needs and monitored closely by their healthcare providers.

Lifestyle changes for chronic diseases

Making lifestyle changes can help reduce the risk of developing chronic diseases or managing symptoms if a chronic condition has already been diagnosed. Healthy lifestyle changes include:

1. **Balanced Diet**

    Incorporating lifestyle changes such as a balanced diet, regular physical activity, and stress management is crucial for individuals with chronic diseases. The Rice Diet, which emphasizes whole grains and plant-based foods, can help reduce inflammation and improve heart health.

2. **Exercise**

    Engaging in regular physical activity is a vital lifestyle change for individuals with chronic diseases. It not only improves heart health, reduces high blood pressure, and boosts overall energy levels but also reduces the risk of chronic disease progression.

    Adopting both cardiovascular exercise and strength training helps to mitigate symptoms and maintain a healthy body weight. It is also recommended to include personalized exercise routines and incorporate social activities to promote adherence and enjoyment.

3. **Stress management**

   Lifestyle Changes for Chronic Diseases often involve stress management techniques like deep breathing exercises, mindfulness meditation, or yoga. These techniques can lower cortisol levels and activate the parasympathetic nervous system, which can have a positive impact on chronic conditions such as hypertension, diabetes, or asthma.

   Engaging in these practices regularly can improve quality of life, increase resilience and decrease the risk of developing other health complications. Incorporating stress management techniques is a simple yet effective way to manage chronic diseases and promote overall wellness.

4. **Quitting Smoking**

   Quitting smoking is one such change and plays a critical role in managing symptoms and reducing the risk of developing further health issues. It is a well-known fact that smoking can worsen the symptoms associated with chronic diseases such as heart disease, diabetes, and respiratory illnesses.

By taking the initiative to quit smoking, individuals can improve their health outcomes and lead healthier lives. Studies have shown that quitting smoking can significantly reduce the burden of chronic disease in everyday life, leading to a more comfortable and fulfilling existence.

5. Limiting alcohol consumption

Limiting alcohol consumption is considered one of the important lifestyle changes for individuals with chronic diseases such as liver disease, heart disease, diabetes, and hypertension.

Healthcare professionals strongly advise their patients to limit their alcohol intake or eliminate it from their lifestyle completely. Alcohol can exacerbate the symptoms of these chronic diseases and may lead to further complications or poor health outcomes.

6. Getting Enough Sleep

Getting enough sleep is paramount for individuals with chronic diseases. Studies have found that inadequate sleep can lead to inflammation and an increased risk of developing cardiovascular disease or stroke, along with emotional issues such as depression and anxiety.

More than seven hours of sleep per night is recommended for adults. If insomnia occurs, consulting a healthcare provider should be the first step to prevent further health issues from developing.

7. **Managing Medications**

   It is important to take medications as prescribed by a healthcare provider for chronic diseases. It should also be noted that some supplements and herbs may have interactions with certain medications, so consulting a healthcare professional before using natural remedies is necessary.

   Additionally, individuals should not stop taking any medication without their doctor's approval, as this can cause further health issues.

8. **Regular Check-Ups**

   Regular check-ups are necessary for getting an accurate diagnosis and tracking the progression of chronic diseases. These appointments should include physical examinations, blood tests, and other diagnostic tests that can help to monitor health status.

   By following up regularly with a healthcare team, individuals can get individualized care and receive information on lifestyle changes that may be beneficial in managing their condition.

Making lifestyle changes for chronic diseases can be daunting, but it does not have to be a difficult process. By educating yourself about the different options available and engaging in activities that promote overall health and well-being, individuals with chronic diseases can improve their quality of life and reduce the burden on them.

What Is a Rice Diet?

The Rice Diet, created by Dr. Walter Kempner at Duke University in the 1930s, was initially designed as a treatment for high blood pressure. Dr. Kempner discovered that a simple diet centered around rice and fruits significantly reduced blood pressure, inspiring the development of the Rice Diet as a structured program.

Over the years, the Rice Diet has evolved to become a comprehensive program for improving overall health and well-being. The diet is based on whole, unprocessed foods that are low in fat and cholesterol but high in fiber, vitamins, and minerals. This approach to eating can help to reduce inflammation in the body, lower blood pressure, and reduce the risk of heart disease and diabetes.

The Rice Diet emphasizes the importance of plant-based foods as a primary source of nutrition. The diet encourages the consumption of fruits, vegetables, whole grains, and legumes, which are rich in nutrients and fiber. These plant-based foods can help to reduce the risk of chronic diseases and promote weight loss.

Portion control and moderation are also prominent features of the Rice Diet. While the diet includes foods that are high in starch, such as rice and potatoes, these foods are consumed in moderate amounts and balanced with protein-rich foods such as fish and chicken. By following this approach to eating, you can consume a nutritionally balanced diet while still promoting weight loss and improving your health.

The Rice Diet also allows for flexibility in food choices, making it easier to sustain long-term healthy eating habits. Unlike many strict diets that require you to eliminate entire food groups or adhere to specific meal plans, the Rice Diet allows you to choose from a variety of foods.

In our upcoming sections, we will explore the benefits of the Rice Diet in more detail and discuss how you can incorporate this diet into your daily life. By following the Rice Diet, you can take control of your health and transform your well-being.

Scientific Evidence Supporting the Rice Diet

Below are some of the scientific evidence supporting the health benefits of following the Rice Diet:

Hypertension

Dr. Kempner initially designed the Rice Diet to treat malignant hypertension—extremely high blood pressure not responsive to regular treatment. One of his earliest studies included over 500 patients diagnosed with this condition. The findings were groundbreaking at the time. Around 60% of the participants experienced a significant reduction in both systolic and diastolic blood pressure. For some, the Rice Diet allowed discontinuation of medications entirely.

Additionally, contemporary researchers examining low-sodium diets often cite the Rice Diet as a notable example of how dramatic dietary intervention can alter biomarkers for hypertension. The low-sodium approach combined with calorie control helps reduce water retention and strain on the cardiovascular system, which translates to consistent blood pressure reduction.

Diabetes and Blood Sugar Regulation

Beyond blood pressure control, the Rice Diet's emphasis on low-fat, plant-based foods also benefits individuals with diabetes or insulin resistance. While the high-carbohydrate component might seem counterintuitive for diabetes management, the diet includes mainly complex carbohydrates, which are digested slowly and contribute to stable blood sugar levels.

A recent study evaluated the impact of a low-fat, rice-based diet on glycemic control. Participants with type 2 diabetes followed a modified version of the Rice Diet for 12 weeks. The results showed improved fasting blood sugar and hemoglobin A1c levels, suggesting better long-term glucose regulation. This aligns with earlier observations from Kempner's era, where patients often experienced reductions in medication requirements or complete remission of symptoms when following the diet strictly.

Obesity and Weight Loss

Effective weight loss is another hallmark of the Rice Diet. A key factor is its focus on calorie control. Studies have validated that diets low in dietary fat and animal protein significantly reduce caloric density while promoting satiety.

One notable study published in The Journal of the American Dietetic Association followed a group of obese participants who adhered to the Rice Diet for six months. The average weight loss across the cohort was 63 pounds, with participants reporting improvements in blood pressure, cholesterol levels, and overall well-being. This outcome rivals even highly restrictive modern weight-loss diets, yet with additional benefits for long-term heart health.

Kidney Disease

Dr. Kempner's early work also highlighted the effectiveness of the Rice Diet in managing kidney disease. High-protein diets are known to increase kidney workload, causing further damage in individuals with compromised kidney function. By drastically reducing protein intake, the Rice Diet helps alleviate strain on the kidneys, preventing further decline.

A retrospective analysis of patients with chronic kidney disease dating back to Kempner's original research demonstrated stabilization in many patients' creatinine and blood urea nitrogen levels. Though these results might not always match the advances provided by modern drug therapy, they underscore the diet's potential role as part of a comprehensive treatment plan.

Modern Interpretations and Future Research

While the original Rice Diet has evolved, its scientific foundations remain robust. Many of its principles align with modern plant-based eating patterns, such as the DASH (Dietary Approaches to Stop Hypertension) diet and the Mediterranean diet, which the medical community widely endorses.

Newer research seeks to explore the longer-term sustainability of rice-based dietary interventions and their applications to broader populations. Questions include how individuals with less stringent health needs—such as moderate obesity or prediabetes—respond to the diet and whether its benefits can be replicated when slightly less restrictive.

Further, the inclusion of whole grain rice over white rice, as well as the addition of legumes for protein supplementation, appears to carry potential for enhancing both nutrient content and health outcomes.

The Rice Diet represents more than a historical approach to combating chronic illness; it serves as a foundation for understanding the power of dietary interventions in achieving better health. Research spanning years, from Dr. Kempner's early pioneering studies to recent clinical trials, supports its effectiveness for conditions like hypertension, diabetes, and obesity.

By focusing on the simplicity and nutrient density of plant-based foods, the Rice Diet opens the door for addressing some of the world's most pressing health challenges. Although modern reinterpretations may update or adjust its specifics, its scientific backing remains clear—what you eat has a profound impact on your well-being.

Principles of the Rice Diet

The Rice Diet is based on a set of principles that emphasize the consumption of whole, plant-based foods and the adoption of a healthy lifestyle. Here are the principles of the Rice Diet:

1. **Eat mostly whole, plant-based foods**

   The Rice Diet emphasizes the inclusion of whole, plant-based foods in one's diet, including an array of fruits, vegetables, whole grains, legumes, and nuts. These nutrient-dense foods are naturally low in saturated fat and cholesterol while being high in fiber, vitamins, and minerals.

Consuming a predominantly plant-based diet has been linked to numerous health benefits, including lowered risk of chronic diseases such as heart disease and certain cancers. By focusing on whole, plant-based foods, the Rice Diet promotes optimal health and well-being.

2. **Choose low-sodium foods**

The Rice Diet is a well-known approach to healthy eating that prioritizes foods low in sodium. Sodium is a mineral that can spike blood pressure and increase the risk of heart problems, such as stroke and heart attack.

By emphasizing low-sodium foods, the Rice Diet aims to protect its followers from these risks. Such foods include fresh fruits and vegetables, lean proteins, and whole grains. These options are not only low in sodium but also nutrient-dense, providing essential vitamins and minerals for overall health. By choosing these low-sodium options, followers of the Rice Diet can promote their health simply and effectively.

3. **Avoid high-fat and processed foods**

   Another key principle of the Rice Diet is to avoid high-fat and processed foods, such as fried foods, sweets, and processed meats. These types of foods are loaded with unhealthy fats, calories, and sodium, which can raise the risk of obesity, heart disease, and other chronic illnesses.

   Instead, the Rice Diet recommends incorporating whole grains, fruits, vegetables, and lean proteins into your diet. By making these healthier food choices, individuals can improve their overall health and reduce their risk of chronic disease. So, it is crucial to revamp eating habits and take the necessary steps towards leading a healthy lifestyle.

4. **Emphasize healthy fats**

   The Rice Diet advocates a low-fat diet that is rich in healthy fats. Specifically, it encourages the consumption of avocados, nuts, and seeds, which are sources of monounsaturated and polyunsaturated fats that have been shown to improve cholesterol levels and heart health.

   Rather than eliminating fats from one's diet, the Rice Diet promotes the inclusion of healthy fats that provide numerous health benefits. By emphasizing the importance of healthy fats, this diet can help individuals achieve a balanced and nutritious eating plan that supports overall well-being.

5. **Limit animal protein**

   The Rice Diet also limits the consumption of animal proteins, such as red meats and dairy products. These foods are high in saturated fat and cholesterol, which can raise one's risk of various chronic diseases.

   By limiting these animal proteins, individuals can reduce their risk of illness while still getting an adequate amount of protein from plant-based sources. Furthermore, choosing a mostly plant-based diet can help reduce one's carbon footprint, making it a win-win for overall health and the planet.

6. **Focus on calorie restriction**

   The Rice Diet focuses on calorie restriction and portion control, meaning that followers should aim to consume fewer calories than they expend. This approach helps individuals reach a healthy weight while avoiding nutritional deficiencies.

   Additionally, caloric restriction has been linked to numerous health benefits, including improved longevity and reduced risk of chronic diseases. So, it is important to be mindful of one's caloric intake and to focus on consuming nutrient-rich foods in the right amounts.

7. **Engage in regular physical activity**

   It is important to engage in regular physical activity. Exercise has been linked to numerous health benefits, such as improved cardiovascular health and lower risk of chronic disease. So, individuals should aim to get at least 30 minutes of exercise each day to promote overall well-being.

8. **Manage stress**

   Finally, followers of the Rice Diet should make an effort to manage their stress levels. Stress has been linked to a variety of health concerns, including weight gain, heart disease, and depression. So, it is important to take time for self-care and to practice mindfulness techniques that can help manage stress levels.

By following the principles of the Rice Diet and engaging in healthy lifestyle behaviors, individuals can improve their overall health and well-being. So, it is important to take the necessary steps toward leading a healthier life.

Benefits of the Rice Diet

The rice diet is a plant-based, low-fat, and high-carbohydrate diet that provides numerous health benefits. Here are the benefits of the rice diet:

1. **Weight loss**

   The Rice Diet program offers several benefits for individuals seeking sustainable weight loss. One of its main advantages is providing a low-fat, plant-based diet that is high in fiber and essential nutrients. This approach has been proven to promote weight loss while also improving overall health.

   Additionally, the program's emphasis on calorie restriction and healthy eating habits ensures long-term success. Moreover, the Rice Diet may help manage certain health conditions, such as high blood pressure, diabetes, and heart disease, as it promotes a healthy lifestyle through diet and exercise.

2. **Lower blood pressure**

   A rice diet is an effective option for individuals with hypertension as it emphasizes low-sodium foods and high-fiber foods. This diet has been proven to lower blood pressure levels. Consuming low-sodium foods helps maintain healthy blood pressure levels, while high-fiber foods help reduce cholesterol levels, which in turn decreases the risk of cardiovascular disease. The benefits of the rice diet make it an ideal option for people looking to regulate their blood pressure and live a healthy life.

3. **Lower cholesterol levels**

   The rice diet has been known to significantly improve cholesterol levels and promote better heart health. This low-fat, plant-based diet is inherently low in saturated fats and cholesterol. By incorporating the rice diet into one's lifestyle, individuals can effectively reduce their risk of heart disease and other related conditions. The diet is rich in essential nutrients, including fiber, minerals, and vitamins, making it an excellent choice for those looking to adopt a healthier lifestyle.

4. **Improved blood sugar control**

   The rice diet has been proven to effectively improve blood sugar control, making it an ideal dietary intervention for individuals with diabetes. By consuming a diet that is low in salt, fat, and refined carbohydrates, while high in complex carbohydrates such as rice, patients can experience significant reductions in their blood sugar levels. This has been attributed to the high fiber content of complex carbohydrates, which slows the absorption of sugar from the bloodstream.

5. **Increased fiber intake**

   The benefits of the rice diet don't just stop at its rich fiber content. Its high fiber intake also aids in lowering cholesterol levels, maintaining healthy blood sugar levels, and managing weight. Additionally, the diet is rich in essential vitamins and minerals that are necessary for optimal health.

It's also a low-sodium and low-fat diet, making it an ideal option for those looking to improve their overall well-being. A rice diet is truly a holistic approach to healthy living, and its benefits extend beyond just digestion and cancer prevention.

6. **Nutrient-dense diet**

In addition to being nutrient-dense, the Rice Diet has been praised for its numerous health benefits. Studies have shown that following such a diet can lead to weight loss, improved heart health, and a reduced risk of chronic diseases such as diabetes, high blood pressure, and cancer.

Additionally, the consumption of whole grains like brown rice has been linked to improved digestion and a lower risk of gastrointestinal issues. By focusing on whole, nutrient-rich foods, the Rice Diet promotes overall health and well-being.

7. **Reduced inflammation**

The benefits of the rice diet go beyond weight loss. Indeed, one of the most significant advantages is its potential to reduce inflammation in the body, an underlying factor in many chronic diseases such as heart disease, diabetes, and cancer.

This is because the rice diet is predominantly plant-based and low in processed foods, which tend to be high in sugar, unhealthy fats, and sodium. Research has shown that following a low-inflammatory diet can lower the risk of chronic diseases and improve overall health.

8. Lifestyle modifications

Lifestyle modifications like regular exercise, stress management, and community support play a crucial role in maintaining the long-term health benefits of the Rice Diet. Therefore, this diet is a smart choice for individuals seeking a sustainable and effective approach to improving their health.

The Rice Diet offers multiple benefits for individuals seeking to improve their health. By following this diet, people can experience a reduction in blood pressure and cholesterol levels, which in turn leads to a decreased risk of heart disease and stroke. Moreover, the diet emphasizes the intake of nutrient-dense foods that provide the body with essential vitamins and minerals.

Overall, the rice diet can help individuals achieve sustainable weight loss and lead a healthy lifestyle while providing numerous other health benefits such as improved heart health, blood sugar control, and reduced inflammation.

Disadvantages of the Rice Diet

While the rice diet provides numerous health benefits, it is important to consider the potential disadvantages before starting the program. Here are the disadvantages of the Rice Diet:

1. **Limited food options**

    The Rice Diet, while effective for weight loss, can be difficult to maintain for individuals who are accustomed to a diverse range of foods. The limited food options can quickly become monotonous and unappetizing, leading to a higher likelihood of falling off the diet.

    Furthermore, the diet's high carbohydrate intake may not be suitable for everyone, such as those with diabetes or other health conditions that require controlled blood sugar levels. The lack of protein in the diet can also be a concern for individuals who require a higher protein intake for muscle maintenance and repair.

2. **Reduction in energy levels**

    The Rice Diet, while effective in weight loss and reducing blood pressure, does have some disadvantages. The initial phase involves calorie restriction, which can lead to notable reductions in energy levels and feelings of fatigue.

As calorie intake is limited, the body shifts into a state where it burns stored fat for energy, resulting in temporary dips in blood sugar levels that can exacerbate fatigue. Additionally, the strict dietary limitations of the Rice Diet can result in nutrient deficiencies, particularly for those consuming it for extended periods.

3. Risk of nutrient deficiencies

While the rice diet can lead to initial weight loss and improve certain health markers, strict adherence to this diet can result in nutrient deficiencies. This is particularly concerning if the individual does not consume a variety of whole, plant-based foods.

Nutrient deficiencies can manifest in various ways, including fatigue, weakness, and impaired cognitive function. Additionally, restrictive diets like this may be unsustainable, leading to a cycle of weight regain and further health complications.

4. Lack of social feasibility

While the Rice Diet has been touted for its health benefits, it may not be socially feasible. This is because the diet limits an individual's ability to eat out or attend social events that involve food, leading to feelings of isolation and exclusion. Not being able to eat with family and friends can also lead to social and emotional strain.

5. **Not suitable for everyone**

    Despite its potential benefits for weight loss and treating certain medical conditions, the rice diet may not be suitable for everyone. Individuals with celiac disease or gluten intolerance cannot follow the rice diet, as some foods included in the diet contain gluten.

    Additionally, the diet may not provide enough nutrients for pregnant or breastfeeding women, children, or athletes. Those with diabetes must also be cautious when following the rice diet, as it may cause blood sugar levels to fluctuate.

    Furthermore, the diet is not recommended for those with a history of eating disorders, as it may trigger unhealthy behaviors. Consultation with a healthcare professional is essential before starting the rice diet to ensure that it is appropriate for an individual's specific needs and health status.

However, by following the principles of the rice diet, individuals can reap the benefits while avoiding potential drawbacks. It is important to speak with a healthcare provider before starting any new diet or lifestyle program.

Common Challenges and Solutions

The Rice Diet is renowned for its effectiveness in managing chronic health conditions like hypertension, diabetes, and obesity. However, as with any structured eating plan, it comes with its own set of challenges.

Strict dietary restrictions and lifestyle adjustments can feel overwhelming at times. The good news? With mindful strategies, these obstacles can be overcome. Below, we explore common challenges faced by those following the Rice Diet and provide practical solutions to help you stay on track.

1. **Adherence to the Diet's Restrictions**

   Challenge:

   The Rice Diet focuses on low sodium, low fat, and low protein foods, which can feel limiting—especially in today's food culture where processed and high-sodium products dominate. For some, the monotony of eating rice, fruits, and vegetables frequently may lead to cravings or burnout.

   Solution:

Start by diversifying your meals within the diet's guidelines. Incorporate a variety of fruits, vegetables, and rice-based dishes to keep things interesting. Experiment with seasonings like garlic, ginger, lemon, and fresh herbs instead of salt. Spice blends without sodium can also add flavor while keeping you compliant.

Batch-cooking meals can be helpful too. Prepare soups, rice bowls, and fruit salads in advance so you always have something on hand, reducing the temptation to stray. Setting small, manageable goals—like committing to a week at a time—can also make the diet feel less daunting. Celebrate milestones to stay motivated.

If cravings strike, pause and remind yourself why you started the Rice Diet in the first place. Revisit your health goals and visualize how far you've come—it's a great way to strengthen your resolve.

2. **Dining Out While Staying Compliant**

Challenge:

Navigating restaurant menus while adhering to the Rice Diet can be tricky. Many meals are laden with salt, fat, or hidden ingredients that don't fit the guidelines.

Solution:

Before dining out, review the restaurant's menu online if possible. Look for dishes that can be customized, such as steamed vegetables, plain rice, or salads without dressing. Don't be shy about asking the kitchen staff to accommodate your needs—most restaurants can prepare simple, unsalted meals on request.

If eating at someone else's home, communicate your dietary preferences in advance. Offer to bring a dish you can enjoy so there's a guaranteed option for you at the table.

Make it about the experience of socializing and not just the food. Sip on seltzer water, enjoy the company, and focus on staying consistent with your own meal choices, no matter the setting.

3. Finding Suitable Substitutes for Restricted Foods

Challenge:

Many people miss staples like bread, dairy, or high-protein foods when following the Rice Diet. Limited options can leave you wondering what to eat when cravings hit.

Solution:

The key here is finding satisfying swaps. Instead of high-sodium snack foods, try fresh fruit, rice cakes, or homemade unsalted popcorn. Replace processed sauces with homemade salsa or dips made from blended fruits or vegetables. Use sweet potatoes or squash as comforting carb alternatives when rice starts to feel repetitive.

For those concerned about protein intake, add legume-based options like lentils or chickpeas. While traditional Rice Diet plans limit these more than modern interpretations, they can provide variety for those on less restrictive versions of the diet. Just remember to follow portion guidelines.

Keep your pantry stocked with essentials like low-sodium canned vegetables, quick-cooking rice varieties, and fruit cups packed in juice (not syrup). With the right ingredients at arm's length, you'll feel equipped to handle cravings.

4. **Social Situations and Peer Pressure**

   Challenge:

Sticking to the Rice Diet in social situations—like family gatherings, holidays, or parties—can feel challenging. Well-meaning friends and family might even question your choices or encourage you to "cheat just this once."

Solution:

First, stand firm in your decision and communicate your reasons. Saying something as simple as, "I'm following this diet for my health, and it makes me feel great," can go a long way. Most people will respect your commitment when you explain your motivation.

Bring your own dish to gatherings so you can eat confidently and still participate in the meal. For example, a big fruit salad or a vegetable platter can fit both your guidelines and the occasion.

If someone tries to pressure you, redirect the conversation to non-food-related topics. Remember, you have the right to prioritize your health without needing to justify yourself to others.

5. **Maintaining Motivation Over Time**

Challenge:

The results of any diet often come gradually, and it's easy to lose motivation without quick visible changes. Plateaus or moments of discouragement can make it difficult to keep going.

Solution:

Focus on more than just the scale. Track other markers of improvement, such as lower blood pressure, improved energy levels, or better control of blood sugar. Keeping a health journal can help you see the progress you've made—even the small wins.

Surround yourself with a support network. Find others on a similar health journey, whether in person or through online communities. Sharing challenges and successes can keep you accountable and motivated.

Remind yourself that the Rice Diet is not simply about weight loss; it's about improving your overall health. Visualize the long-term benefits to your heart, kidneys, and overall well-being every time you start to waver.

Final Tips for Long-Term Success

The Rice Diet may seem like a big lifestyle change, but with the right mindset and support, it can become a sustainable way of living. Here are some final tips to help you maintain your progress over time:

- ***Engage in Meal Planning:*** Set aside one day a week to plan and prep meals that fit the Rice Diet. Having a clear plan minimizes last-minute decisions that could lead to unhealthy choices.
- ***Celebrate Non-Food Rewards:*** Treat yourself to non-food rewards for sticking to the diet—such as a new book, a fitness class, or even a relaxing day off.

- ***Be Kind to Yourself:*** Slip-ups happen. Don't be discouraged by a single misstep. What matters most is consistency over time, not perfection every moment.

By recognizing and addressing these challenges proactively, you set yourself up for long-term success. The Rice Diet may require adjustments and dedication, but with the right strategies, you'll find it easier to stay the course and reap its many health benefits. You've got this!

The 5-Step Guide to Getting Started on the Rice Diet

If you're looking to lose weight or simply live a healthier lifestyle, the rice diet might be the perfect solution for you. This low-fat, low-sodium, and low-calorie diet has been around for decades and has helped many people achieve their health goals. Here's a 5-step guide to getting started on the rice diet:

Step 1: Consult with a healthcare professional

Before starting the Rice Diet, consulting with a healthcare professional is a vital first step. Dietary changes, especially those as structured and restrictive as the Rice Diet, can have significant effects on your body, so it's crucial to ensure it's suitable for your unique health needs. A healthcare professional can evaluate your current medical conditions, such as diabetes, hypertension, or kidney issues, and determine whether this approach aligns with your goals and overall well-being.

They might perform a comprehensive assessment, including blood tests, a review of your medical history, and discussions about your lifestyle habits. This helps them identify potential risks, such as nutrient deficiencies, low energy levels, or interactions with existing medications. For instance, the diet's low protein and fat content may not be appropriate for individuals with specific health conditions or nutritional requirements.

Your healthcare provider can also offer tailored advice on safely starting the diet. They may suggest modifications based on your individual needs, such as portion adjustments, supplements to ensure balanced nutrition, or a gradual transition to the plan. With professional guidance, you can reduce risks, set realistic expectations, and establish a foundation for long-term success on the Rice Diet. This step ensures both safety and sustainability.

Step 2: Stock Up on the Essentials

Getting ready for a successful rice diet starts with a well-stocked kitchen. Here are the key foods you'll need to stay on track and enjoy variety along the way:

- ***Brown Rice:*** This will be your go-to carbohydrate source. Nutty, versatile, and packed with fiber, it provides the foundation for your meals.
- ***Fruits:*** Aim for at least three servings a day to add natural sweetness, vitamins, and a burst of color to

your plate. Think apples, berries, oranges, or whichever fruits you love most.
- **Vegetables:** Load up on at least four servings daily. Fresh, leafy greens, crunchy carrots, and roasted squash all bring nutrients and flavor to your dishes. They'll keep your meals balanced and satisfying.
- **Lean Protein:** Include chicken, fish, tofu, or other lean options to power you through your day. These proteins help you feel full and support your body's needs.
- **Low-Fat Dairy:** Opt for skim milk or yogurt to round out your diet with calcium and protein. These make great snacks or additions to your meals.

By having these essentials on hand, you'll always be ready to whip up a delicious, healthy meal that keeps you moving closer to your goals!

Step 3: Establish Your Meal Plan

With your essentials ready, it's time to create a meal plan that works for you. A well-structured plan will keep you both nourished and energized. Here are some tips to get you started:

1. **Stick to Regular Meals and Snacks:** Aim for three small, balanced meals and two healthy snacks each day to keep your energy levels steady and avoid hunger.
2. **Craft Your Meals with Care:** A typical rice diet meal might feature:

- 1/2 cup of brown rice as your carbohydrate base.
- 1/2 cup of vegetables for a variety of nutrients and flavors.
- 3 ounces of lean protein, like chicken or fish, to help you stay satisfied and meet your nutritional needs.
3. ***Simple and Satisfying Snacks:*** Snacks are a chance to recharge in between meals. Reach for:
    - A small piece of fruit for natural sweetness and vitamins.
    - 1/2 cup of low-fat yogurt, offering a creamy, protein-packed treat.

Planning your meals ahead ensures you stay organized, maintain portion control, and enjoy every bite while moving closer to your health goals. Stay flexible and focus on variety to keep things interesting!

Step 4: Gradually Introduce Rice

Easing into the rice diet is key to setting yourself up for success. By starting slow, your body has time to adjust, and you can avoid any discomfort along the way. Here's how to gradually make rice an essential part of your meals:

- *Week 1:* Begin by replacing just **one meal a day** with a rice diet meal. You can choose which meal works best for you—breakfast, lunch, or dinner. This gentle

start helps your body acclimate to the new eating pattern.
- *Week 2:* Step it up by swapping out **two meals each day** for rice diet meals. You'll start to notice how light yet satisfying these meals can be as your body gets into the rhythm.
- *Week 3:* Now you're ready to go all in! Replace **three meals a day** with rice diet meals, fully committing to the plan while reaping the benefits of this structured approach to eating.

Throughout these weeks, remember to **start with smaller portions of rice** and gradually build up to **1/2 cup per meal**. This method ensures a smooth transition, reduces the risk of any digestive discomfort, and boosts your chances of sticking with the plan for the long haul.

By allowing your body to adapt step by step, you're setting the foundation for a healthier, balanced lifestyle. Stay patient, trust the process, and celebrate each week's progress—you're doing amazing!

Step 5: Keep track and adjust as needed

Tracking your progress is a crucial part of any successful diet or lifestyle change. It helps you stay accountable and allows you to make tweaks that keep you moving toward your goals. Here are some tips to help you stay on course with the rice diet:

- ***Start a Food Journal:*** Write down everything you eat each day. This practice not only keeps you mindful of your choices but also helps identify patterns or areas for improvement.
- ***Monitor Your Weight:*** Weigh yourself regularly (but not obsessively) to track your weight loss progress. Choose a consistent time and day each week for a clearer picture of your results.
- ***Make Adjustments as Needed:*** Your body might need slight tweaks to stay on the right track. If progress slows, consider refining your meal portions, adding variety to your meals, or incorporating more physical activity into your routine.

By consistently tracking and being flexible with your approach, you'll set yourself up for long-term success. Remember, the goal is sustainable, healthy changes—not quick fixes.

The Three Phases of the Rice Diet

The Rice Diet is a unique weight-loss plan used for decades to help people reach their health goals. The diet consists of three main phases, each designed to further facilitate healthy eating habits and promote long-term success. In this chapter, we'll take a look at the three phases of the Rice Diet and how they work together.

Phase 1 of the Rice Diet: Your Comprehensive Guide

Phase 1 of the rice diet is a short-term, focused phase designed to help you shed unwanted weight, reset your eating habits, and nourish your body from the inside out. With its low-calorie, low-sodium, low-fat, and primarily plant-based approach, Phase 1 paves the way for lasting success. Here's everything you need to know to get started:

<u>Beginner Steps</u>

Phase 1 begins with a clean slate. To get the best results:

- *Eliminate animal products:* This means no meat, dairy, or eggs.

- ***Cut out processed and high-fat foods:*** Say goodbye to sugar, salt, and heavily processed snacks.
- ***Focus on whole, plant-based eating:*** The goal is to simplify your meals with natural, nutrient-dense foods.

Think of this phase as a reset for both your body and lifestyle, helping you shift toward healthier habits.

Foods to Eat

During Phase 1 of the rice diet, your focus will be on whole, minimally processed, plant-based foods. Here's what your diet should include:

- ***Brown Rice:*** The star of the rice diet! High in fiber and low in calories, brown rice is a satisfying and nutritious foundation for your meals.
- ***Vegetables:*** Load up on nutrient-packed, low-calorie veggies. Try options like cabbage, kale, spinach, romaine lettuce, celery, carrots, and bell peppers. These add variety, nutrients, and flavor to every dish.
- ***Fruits:*** Aim for 3–4 servings of fruit daily. Choices like apples, berries, bananas, and pears provide natural sweetness, hydration, and a healthy dose of fiber and vitamins.
- ***Beans and Legumes:*** Lentils, chickpeas, navy beans, and black beans are packed with protein, fiber, and essential nutrients. They also help keep you full and energized.

- ***Soy Products:*** Incorporate tofu, edamame, and soy milk for plant-based protein and variety in your diet.
- ***Beverages:*** Stick to water and unsweetened herbal teas to stay hydrated and support your body's natural detox process.

How Long Does Phase 1 Last?

Phase 1 typically lasts one week, giving your body a chance to adapt to a lower calorie intake and plant-based eating. During this time, aim for fewer than 800 calories per day to create a calorie deficit that promotes rapid weight loss. While this phase is intensive, it's brief and designed to jump-start your progress.

Benefits of Phase 1

Phase 1 of the rice diet isn't just about weight loss—it's about improving your overall well-being. Here are some exciting benefits to look forward to:

- ***Rapid Weight Loss:*** The carefully controlled calorie intake helps you see results quickly.
- ***Improved Health Markers:*** Lower blood pressure, reduced cholesterol levels, and better overall health.
- ***A System Reset:*** Detox your body and break free from unhealthy eating patterns.
- ***Positive Food Relationship:*** Learn to appreciate simple, whole foods and repair your relationship with eating.

Phase 1 of the rice diet is about more than just shedding pounds—it's about laying the groundwork for a healthier future. By focusing on a plant-based, low-calorie diet filled with nutrient-dense foods, you'll cleanse your system, boost your nutrition, and reset your habits.

Take this week as an opportunity to commit to yourself. Stick to these guidelines, listen to your body, and celebrate each step forward. You're setting the stage for positive, lasting change!

Phase 2 of the Rice Diet: Understanding the Process

Phase 2 of the rice diet is an extension of Phase 1 and typically lasts two to six weeks. This phase allows for a more extended variety of foods and aims to continue healthy weight loss sustainably. Here is what you need to know about Phase 2 of the rice diet:

Introduction of Foods

In Phase 2, some foods that were restricted in Phase 1 are reintroduced in small amounts. These include:

- *Whole grains:* Whole wheat bread, whole-grain pasta, quinoa, and oatmeal provide a good source of fiber, vitamins, and minerals.
- *Lean protein:* Fish, chicken, turkey, and eggs are reintroduced for their protein content. Be sure to

choose low-fat and low-sodium options for optimal health benefits
- **Low-fat dairy:** Skim milk, low-fat cheese, and Greek yogurt are included for their protein and calcium content.
- **Snacks:** Snacks like unsalted nuts, hummus, and air-popped popcorn in moderation can help satisfy cravings without compromising weight loss goals.

Portion Sizes

While Phase 2 does allow for the introduction of some foods previously restricted in Phase 1, portion sizes are still essential. Limiting portion sizes to the recommended amounts is crucial to maintaining healthy weight loss.

Planning Meals

Phase 2 of the rice diet still emphasizes planning meals ahead of time to ensure proper nutrient intake and portion control. Meal prepping and planning is still a key component of weight loss success in Phase 2.

Incorporating Exercise

Exercise is an essential part of a healthy lifestyle and weight loss. In Phase 2 of the rice diet, it is recommended to start incorporating exercise into your routine gradually. Brisk walks, yoga, swimming, and strength training are excellent activities to get started with.

Continued Progress Tracking

Tracking progress is key to continued success on the rice diet. Phase 2 encourages continued record-keeping of food intake, exercise, and weight loss progress to remain on track and adjust as needed.

Phase 2 of the rice diet is an expansion of Phase 1, allowing for the reintroduction of some foods while still emphasizing portion control, meal planning, and exercise. Continued progress tracking remains crucial to achieving weight loss goals and overall health improvements.

Phase 3 of the Rice Diet: Lifestyle Change and Maintenance

Phase 3 of the rice diet is the long-term maintenance phase after completing Phases 1 and 2. This phase focuses on maintaining healthy food choices, physical activity, and overall wellness for long-term success. Here's what you need to know:

Maintenance Goals

The primary goal of Phase 3 is to maintain the weight loss achieved in the previous phases while also focusing on overall wellness. This involves making long-term lifestyle changes and healthy choices that are sustainable over time.

Foods to Eat

Phase 3 allows for more flexibility in food choices while still emphasizing healthy, whole foods. Dieters should focus on choosing foods that are low in saturated fat, added sugars, and sodium.

Some recommended foods include:

- *Whole grains:* Brown rice, whole wheat bread, quinoa, and whole-grain pasta provide a good source of fiber, vitamins, and minerals.
- *Lean protein:* Fish, chicken, turkey, and eggs are optimal protein sources when chosen in their low-fat forms.
- *Low-fat dairy:* Skim milk, low-fat cheese, and Greek yogurt can provide additional protein and calcium.
- Fruits and vegetables: A variety of fruits and vegetables in different colors should make up a significant portion of the diet.
- *Soy products:* Tofu, soy milk, and edamame remain great sources of plant-based protein.

Portion Control

In Phase 3, portion control continues to be an essential part of maintaining healthy habits. Practice mindful eating and listen to your body's hunger and fullness cues.

Exercise

Regular exercise should be a staple in Phase 3 to maintain weight loss and overall health. Dieters should aim to incorporate at least 30 minutes of physical activity each day, such as walking, biking, or strength training.

Continued Progress Tracking

Tracking progress is still key to maintaining success during Phase 3. Dieters should continue to track food intake, exercise, and weight loss progress to stay on track and make adjustments if necessary.

Benefits of Phase 3

Phase 3 of the rice diet emphasizes making long-term lifestyle changes and focuses on overall health and wellness. Maintaining healthy eating habits, regular physical activity, and ongoing progress tracking can help dieters maintain weight loss and improve their overall health.

Phase 3 of the rice diet is the long-term maintenance phase that focuses on making healthy lifestyle changes and maintaining weight loss. Eating a balanced diet rich in whole foods, practicing portion control, regular exercise and ongoing progress tracking are the keys to success during Phase 3.

Measuring Portion Sizes

When preparing your meals, you must be very particular with serving sizes to ensure the success of your diet. Here are some basic guidelines:

- One fruit is one cup of cut fruit or one piece of medium-sized fruit.
- One cup of starch is one-half cup of cooked rice/beans, one-half cup of cooked pasta, oatmeal, quinoa, dried beans, or one slice of bread.
- One vegetable equals one-half cup cooked or one cup uncooked.
- One dairy equals 1/2 cup cottage cheese, 1 cup low-fat yogurt, or 1 cup milk.

Determining a portion size for lean protein foods is more challenging. If you have a scale, then one portion of lean protein is equal to around 3 oz. of skinless chicken, lean beef, or fish.

You can also estimate by cutting the protein into an approximate size compared with common objects. One portion of meat (3 oz.) is the size of a deck of cards. One portion of the fish is the size of a checkbook.

You can eat either white or brown rice based on your personal preferences. However, brown rice is seen as being higher in fiber and other nutrients since it has not been processed and still retains its shell. On the other hand, it takes longer to cook since you will have to soak it in water for twenty minutes.

In addition, you can make the rice more palatable by cooking it with herbs and spices. For instance, you can heat some chopped onions and minced garlic and add them to cooked rice. Then, sprinkle some paprika and parsley to taste.

To ensure that you are staying within your allowed calorie limit, you can use calorie counter apps and websites. Many of these are available to download or use for free. Some of these have features that allow them to sync with fitness tracking devices, so you can download the data into their exercise log.

Foods to Eat in the Rice Diet

The Rice Diet is a plant-based, low-fat, and high-carbohydrate diet that emphasizes whole, nutrient-dense foods. Here are the foods that individuals can eat in the Rice Diet:

1. **Fruits**

    The Rice Diet promotes a healthy lifestyle by suggesting a variety of fruits to incorporate into one's diet. Berries, such as blueberries and raspberries, are rich in antioxidants and can reduce inflammation.

    Oranges are packed with vitamin C and can improve heart health. Grapes contain resveratrol, which may reduce the risk of certain cancers. Apples are full of fiber and can aid in digestion. Bananas are a good source of potassium and can help regulate blood pressure. Including a variety of these fruits can not only satisfy one's sweet cravings but also improve overall health.

2. Vegetables

The Rice Diet promotes the consumption of a variety of nutritious vegetables to enhance overall health and wellness. Spinach, kale, broccoli, peppers, and carrots are among the highly recommended veggies that are rich in essential nutrients such as vitamins A, C, and K, fiber, and antioxidants.

These vegetables aid in digestion, reduce inflammation, and promote weight loss. Consuming these foods as part of a well-balanced diet can lead to improved overall health and a decreased risk of chronic diseases like heart disease and type 2 diabetes.

3. Whole grains

Including brown rice, quinoa, barley, and oats in one's diet is essential for a healthy lifestyle, particularly when following the Rice Diet. These whole grains provide plenty of vitamins, minerals, and antioxidants that can help prevent chronic diseases such as heart disease and diabetes.

4. **Legumes**

   For those following the Rice Diet, incorporating legumes such as beans, lentils, peas, and other plant-based sources of protein and fiber can be an excellent choice. These foods are nutritionally rich and can help to support good health, as they are low in fat and calories while being high in essential vitamins, minerals, and antioxidants.

   Additionally, legumes are a great option for those looking to maintain a healthy weight, as they can help to promote feelings of fullness and satisfaction after meals. By including legumes in their diets, those following the Rice Diet can feel confident that they are getting the nourishment they need to stay healthy and thrive.

5. **Nuts and seeds**

   Almonds, cashews, chia seeds, flaxseeds, and other nuts and seeds are highly recommended foods in the Rice Diet due to their impressive nutritional values. These foods are excellent sources of protein and healthy fats, which are essential for maintaining a healthy body.

   For instance, almonds are rich in vitamin E, magnesium, and fiber, while cashews are a great source of zinc, copper, and iron. Chia seeds and flaxseeds, on the other hand, are abundant in omega-3 fatty acids, fiber, and antioxidants.

Consuming these nuts and seeds as part of the Rice Diet can provide numerous health benefits such as reducing the risk of heart disease and diabetes while promoting healthy digestion and weight management.

6. **Lean protein**

In the Rice Diet plan, individuals can enjoy a range of lean protein sources that are both delicious and nutritious. Such sources include skinless chicken, turkey, fish, and low-fat dairy products. These lean protein sources provide essential amino acids, vitamins, and minerals needed for a balanced diet.

7. **Healthy fats**

The Rice Diet emphasizes the consumption of healthy fats, including avocados and olive oil, in moderation. These foods are excellent sources of monounsaturated and polyunsaturated fats, which can promote heart health by reducing cholesterol levels and inflammation.

Avocados also provide essential vitamins and minerals such as potassium and vitamin K, making them a nutritious addition to any diet. Additionally, consuming healthy fats can help individuals feel fuller for longer periods, aiding in weight loss efforts. Overall, understanding the critical components of the Rice Diet is integral for achieving optimal health and nutrition.

Including these foods in one's diet can help to promote long-term health and wellness, while also supporting weight loss goals. By following the Rice Diet, individuals can enjoy a variety of nutritious meals that are both delicious and satisfying. With proper guidance, discipline, and dedication, anyone can achieve their desired nutrition goals using the Rice Diet as a guide.

Foods to Avoid in the Rice Diet

The Rice Diet is a low-fat, plant-based dietary program that limits certain foods to promote weight loss and overall health. Here are the foods to avoid in the Rice Diet:

Processed foods

The Rice Diet emphasizes the importance of avoiding processed foods to achieve optimal health. This includes fried foods, highly-sugared candies, and other high-fat snacks. These types of processed foods are known to harm overall health and can lead to weight gain, diabetes, and other chronic health conditions.

By avoiding these processed foods and instead focusing on whole, nutrient-dense foods, individuals can improve their health and achieve their weight loss goals on the Rice Diet.

High-fat foods

Red meat, bacon, butter, and full-fat dairy products are considered high-fat foods that are deemed unsuitable for the Rice Diet. These foods contain high amounts of saturated and trans fats, which can lead to a variety of health problems, including high blood pressure, heart disease, and obesity.

Eating a diet rich in fruits, vegetables, whole grains, and lean protein instead of these high-fat foods can improve overall health and reduce the risk of chronic diseases. Therefore, individuals following the Rice Diet are advised to avoid these high-fat foods to achieve optimal results.

High-sodium foods

In the Rice Diet, it is recommended to avoid consuming high-sodium foods like canned soups, chips, and processed meats. These foods are known to contain excessive amounts of sodium which can lead to high blood pressure and other health problems.

To maintain a healthy diet, it is crucial to opt for low-sodium alternatives and natural sources of nutrients. By avoiding high-sodium foods in the Rice Diet, individuals can have better control over their sodium intake and reap the benefits of a well-balanced and nutritious diet.

Refined carbohydrates

White bread, pasta, and rice are refined carbohydrates that should be limited or avoided in the Rice Diet. These highly processed foods lack important nutrients and can cause spikes in blood sugar levels, leading to cravings and weight gain. Moreover, the refining process strips the grains of their natural fiber, further increasing their glycemic index.

Instead, the Rice Diet promotes the consumption of whole grains, fruits, vegetables, and lean proteins to support optimal health and weight management. By making simple dietary changes, individuals can improve their overall wellness while avoiding the negative consequences of refined carbohydrates.

Sugar-sweetened beverages

Sugar-sweetened beverages are known to be high in calories and sugar, therefore, they are discouraged from the Rice Diet. These types of beverages include energy drinks, fruit juices, and soda.

Consuming these beverages can increase the risk of obesity, type 2 diabetes, and heart disease. On the Rice Diet, individuals are encouraged to choose healthier beverage options such as water, unsweetened tea, and coffee, which can promote weight loss and improve overall health.

Overall, the foods to avoid in the Rice Diet are those that are high in calories, unhealthy fats, sodium, and sugar. By avoiding these foods and emphasizing a plant-based, nutrient-dense, and low-fat diet, individuals can achieve sustainable weight loss and overall health improvements.

Adjusting the Rice Diet for Specific Needs

The rice diet is a flexible and health-focused plan designed to aid weight loss and improve overall well-being. However, certain medical conditions like diabetes, hypertension, or gluten intolerance require thoughtful adjustments to ensure the diet supports individual health needs while remaining effective. Below, you'll find tailored guidance for modifying the rice diet to suit these specific conditions.

Adjusting the Rice Diet for Diabetes

For individuals with diabetes, managing blood sugar levels is a top priority. While the rice diet relies on plant-based carbohydrates like brown rice, which can impact blood sugar, careful planning keeps the diet beneficial and safe.

Practical Tips:

- ***Opt for Low Glycemic Index (GI) Foods:*** Replace or combine brown rice with low-GI alternatives like quinoa or barley. Add fiber-rich vegetables like

spinach or broccoli to slow the absorption of sugars into the bloodstream.
- ***Prioritize Balanced Meals:*** Pair carbs with healthy fats and proteins like avocado, tofu, or grilled chicken to help stabilize blood sugar. For example, combine a small portion of brown rice with sautéed veggies and lean protein.
- ***Monitor Portions:*** Keep rice or grain portions to 1/3 cup per meal to avoid sharp blood sugar spikes. Lean heavily on non-starchy vegetables to bulk up meals.
- ***Include Regular Snacks:*** Incorporate snacks like a handful of almonds, Greek yogurt, or apple slices with peanut butter to maintain steady blood sugar between meals.
- ***Track Blood Sugar:*** Regularly monitor glucose levels after meals to adjust portions or ingredients as needed for better control.

By focusing on nutrient-dense, balanced meals in small portions, diabetics can successfully follow the rice diet while keeping their blood sugar in check.

Adjusting the Rice Diet for Hypertension

For individuals managing high blood pressure, the rice diet's naturally low sodium and plant-based approach align well with health goals. However, some adjustments can further enhance its benefits for heart health.

Practical Tips:

- *Go Sodium-Free:* Completely eliminate table salt, processed foods, and high-sodium condiments like soy sauce. Instead, season dishes with herbs, spices, garlic, or lemon juice.
- *Choose Potassium-Rich Foods:* Add potassium-packed fruits and veggies such as bananas, sweet potatoes, and spinach to help counteract sodium's effects in the body.
- *Use Low-Sodium Protein Options:* Stick to fresh, unprocessed chicken, turkey, beans, and lentils rather than deli meats or canned proteins, which can be high in sodium.
- *Eat Whole Grains Wisely:* Choose unsalted varieties of whole grains like quinoa, barley, or whole wheat pasta to keep sodium intake low.
- *Increase Omega-3s:* Include omega-3-rich foods like salmon, chia seeds, and walnuts, which support heart health and can help lower blood pressure over time.

With mindful ingredient choices and a focus on heart-friendly foods, individuals with hypertension can thrive on the rice diet while safely lowering their blood pressure.

Adjusting the Rice Diet for Gluten Intolerance

Since the rice diet naturally emphasizes gluten-free staples like rice, fruits, and vegetables, it's already a great option for those with gluten intolerance or celiac disease. However, care is required when expanding foods in Phases 2 and 3 to ensure they remain gluten-free.

Practical Tips:

- ***Stick to Gluten-Free Whole Grains:*** Swap out whole wheat bread, pasta, or other gluten-containing grains for quinoa, millet, sorghum, or gluten-free oats.
- ***Read Labels Carefully:*** Be diligent when selecting packaged snacks, sauces, or dairy products to avoid hidden gluten. Look for certified gluten-free labels when in doubt.
- ***Build Meals Around Naturally Gluten-Free Foods:*** Focus on fresh vegetables, brown rice, legumes, soy products, and fresh proteins like chicken, fish, or eggs.
- ***Experiment with Gluten-Free Alternatives:*** Try gluten-free flours like almond or coconut flour to create satisfying alternatives for bread or baked goods if needed.
- ***Avoid Cross-Contamination:*** When preparing meals, use separate utensils and cookware to prevent gluten contamination, especially in shared kitchens.

With careful planning and substitutions, individuals with gluten intolerance can confidently follow the rice diet for weight loss and improved health without compromising their dietary restrictions.

General Considerations for Tailoring the Diet

Now that we've explored specific dietary modifications to the rice diet for certain health conditions, let's dive into some general considerations for tailoring the diet to fit individual needs and preferences.

1. ***Consult a Healthcare Professional:*** Before making any adjustments, discuss your specific health needs and goals with a doctor or dietitian to ensure the rice diet aligns with your condition.
2. ***Listen to Your Body:*** Pay attention to how your body responds to foods and adjustments. If any ingredient triggers discomfort or symptoms, explore alternative options.
3. ***Stay Flexible:*** The rice diet is adaptable to your unique needs. Don't be afraid to make changes while keeping the focus on nutrient-dense, whole foods.

Whether you're managing diabetes, hypertension, gluten intolerance, or another condition, the rice diet can be adjusted to fit your needs while promoting health and weight loss. By making thoughtful substitutions, monitoring portions, and focusing on nutrient-rich foods, you can enjoy the benefits of this diet in a way that works for your body.

Success Stories and Testimonials

William M. O'Barr

William's experience with the Rice Diet is a testament to its effectiveness. Over 3.5 months, he lost 60 pounds, lowered his blood pressure and cholesterol, and stopped relying on medication. The program, which combines fresh, mostly organic foods with exercise and lifestyle education, transformed his relationship with food.

"Cravings disappeared after two or three days without the stimulating effects of salt, oil, and added sugar," he shared. Beyond weight loss, William rediscovered his energy, running through airports and swimming laps with ease. His inspiring story highlights how the Rice Diet fosters not just physical health but also newfound confidence and vitality.

Jean Anspaugh

The Rice Diet's impact on health and weight loss spans decades, inspiring countless transformations. Jean Anspaugh shared how she lost 70 pounds in just four months at the program's residential facility. "One ate rice and fruit and walked," she explained, highlighting the program's disciplined approach.

The Rice Diet not only focused on structured eating but also encouraged active lifestyles and medical supervision. Though the facility has closed, its principles continue to inspire as it showed how dedication to simple, nutrient-dense foods and consistent habits could yield life-changing results. Jean's story proves the power of commitment and a clear goal.

Andrea

Andrea's success with the Rice Diet Program is truly inspiring. When she joined in July 2005, she was ready to make a change. Over a year and a half, Andrea achieved an impressive weight loss of over 80 pounds.

Reflecting on her experience, she shared, "The program gave me the tools I needed to stay on track and transform my health." Andrea managed to keep the weight off with dedication and the support from the Rice Diet principles. Her story shows how sustainable changes and commitment can lead to lasting health improvements and a renewed sense of confidence.

Sample Menus

Here are some sample meals to give you an idea of how to make your own following the Rice Diet guidelines:

- Basic Rice Diet (2 fruits and two starches) = one cup of oatmeal or one slice of toast (starches)
- any two or one cup of strawberries
- one medium banana
- one small orange.

Lacto-Vegetarian Diet

Breakfast

- (one starch, one non-fat dairy, and one fruit) = one slice of toast or one cup of oatmeal
- (starch); one cup of low-fat Greek yogurt or one cup of low-fat milk
- (dairy); one cup of blueberries.

Lunch and Dinner

- (three starches, three vegetables, and one fruit) = 1-1/2 cup cooked beans or rice or three slices of toast

- (starches); 1-1/2 cup steamed asparagus or three cups carrot sticks or celery
- (vegetables); one cup of melon, blueberries, or strawberries or one cup of melon (fruits).

Vegetarian Plus

Breakfast

- (two starches and one fruit) = two slices of toast or one cup of oatmeal
- (starches) and one medium banana or apple (fruit).

Lunch

- (three starches, three vegetables, and one fruit) = 1-1/2 cup of cooked beans
- potatoes
- rice (starches)
- one plum (fruit).

Dinner

- (three proteins, three vegetables, three starches, and one fruit) = three portions of lean
- chicken or fish (proteins)
- 1-1/2 cup cooked rice or potatoes (starches)
- one cup of celery
- one cup of carrots
- one cup of Brussels sprouts (vegetables)

- one cup of pineapple (fruits).

By following these sample menus, the Rice Diet can help individuals achieve a well-rounded diet that is based on whole foods and healthy eating habits. By avoiding processed and high-sugar foods, individuals can achieve sustainable weight loss and overall health improvements.

Sample Recipes

Low-Calorie French Toast

Ingredients:

- 6-8 slices of whole wheat bread (1/2-inch thick is ideal)
- 1 cup nonfat dairy milk
- 1/2 cup orange juice
- 2 tbsp. flour (choose almond flour or coconut flour if available)
- 1 tbsp. sugar (choose coconut sugar if available)
- 1 tbsp. nutritional yeast
- 1/4 tsp. nutmeg
- 1/2 tsp. cinnamon

Instructions:

1. Sift all the dry ingredients into a large bowl.
2. Put all the other ingredients together except the bread and gently mix with a whisk.
3. Preheat a large non-stick skillet to medium heat. Carefully dip bread into the batter mixture.
4. Place on the skillet and cook for about 3 minutes on each side.
5. Repeat the procedure with the remaining bread until the mixture runs out. Any leftover mixture can be refrigerated and used for another batch of bread.
6. It will keep fresh for about 5 days in the fridge. Can be served with cut-up fruits.

Bread Stew

Ingredients:

- vegetable broth, the amount depends on the size of your soup pot
- 1 pc. carrot, chopped
- 1 pc. onion, chopped
- 2 cloves garlic, minced
- 2 stalks of celery, chopped
- 2 cans of 15-ounce, red beans, drained and rinsed
- 1 can of 15-ounce tomatoes, chopped
- 1/4 cup pearled barley
- 1 tsp. oregano leaves, roughly chopped
- freshly ground pepper
- 3 cups fresh spinach, chopped
- 2 cups hearty wheat bread, chopped
- 1 bay leaf

Instructions:

1. Place a small (about a cup or two should be okay to start) amount of the vegetable broth in a large soup pot. Bring the pot to high heat.
2. Add the onion, garlic, celery, and chopped carrot.
3. Wait to boil, stirring occasionally, for about 5 minutes, or until the vegetables have already slightly softened.

4. Add the remaining vegetable broth, then the canned tomatoes, beans, barley, oregano, fresh ground pepper, and bay leaf.
5. Bring the whole pot to a boil and then reduce the heat. Cover the pot and let it sit to cook for about 55 minutes.
6. Add the spinach and cook for an additional 5 minutes. Add in the bread and cook for about 5 minutes more. Serve while still warm.

Note: If you are planning to prepare this bread stew ahead of time, do not add the bread immediately. Reheat the soup again and add until just before serving. For the best soup texture, a hearty Artisan-type bread that is about 1-2 days old works deliciously in this recipe.

Try not to use soft bread as it does not hold its shape well when incorporated into the stew. Small red beans can be used in this recipe, but this could also be made with other types of beans, such as white or black. Pre-soak the beans in water before cooking to shorten the cooking time.

Garbanzo Stew

Ingredients:

- 4 cups vegetable broth
- 2 cans of 15-ounce, garbanzo beans
- 2 tbsp tahini
- 1 pc onion, chopped
- 1 tsp fresh garlic, minced
- 1 pound mushrooms, sliced
- 1-1/2 cups shredded green cabbage
- 1 tsp cumin, ground
- 1/4 tsp coriander, ground
- 1 large roasted red bell pepper, sliced into thick strips
- 1-2 tsp chili-garlic sauce
- 1/2 cup fresh parsley, chopped
- 1/4 cup fresh cilantro, chopped
- 1/4 cup fresh dill, chopped
- 1/4 cup fresh chives, chopped
- 2 tbsp freshly squeezed lemon juice
- sea salt to taste

Instructions:

1. Preheat a large soup pot on low heat.
2. In the large soup pot, lightly saute the onion and garlic using about 1-2 tablespoons of vegetable broth.
3. Stir frequently until the onions soften and turn translucent.

4. Pour in the remaining broth and wait for it to boil.
5. Add the cabbage, coriander, cumin, and mushrooms while stirring.
6. Put the cover, lower the heat, and allow it to simmer for 10-15 minutes.
7. Pour the garbanzos can with juice into a blender.
8. Add the tahini and blend until smooth.
9. Get the remaining can of garbanzo beans, drain, and rinse.
10. Add both the processed beans and the whole beans into the soup pot.
11. Add in as well the roasted red pepper and chili garlic sauce.
12. Bring the pot to a low boil by reducing the heat.
13. Cover and let it simmer for around 40-45 minutes.
14. Add the fresh herbs and lemon juice then simmer again for an additional 15 minutes.
15. Season with a dash of sea salt before serving, if desired.

Tilapia Jasmine Rice

Ingredients:

- 1/2 cup Jasmine rice, uncooked
- 2 pcs Tilapia filets (about 6 ounces each)
- 3/4 cups of water
- 1-1/2 tsp butter
- 1/4 cup fat-free Italian salad dressing
- 1/4 tsp ground cumin
- 1/4 tsp seafood seasoning
- 1/4 tsp fresh ground pepper
- 1/8 tsp salt

Instructions:

1. Preheat a small saucepan to medium heat.
2. Combine the rice, butter, and water in the saucepan and bring to a boil.
3. Immediately reduce the heat to low after boiling.
4. Cover the saucepan and let it simmer until the rice is cooked.
5. You will know it is cooked if the grains have risen and are already tender.
6. Let it simmer for around 15 to 20 minutes, checking towards the latter parts to make sure the rice won't burn.
7. For best results, turn the heat to a really low setting.
8. Add a bit of water if necessary.

9. Meanwhile, mix all the seasonings and sprinkle them all over the tilapia filet.
10. Put an Italian salad dressing on a large skillet and heat, stirring frequently.
11. When the dressing is hot enough, add in the filets and cook until it flakes easily.
12. Cook for about 3-4 minutes on each side. When done, transfer to a plate and serve with the rice.

Yellow Rice

Ingredients:

- 1/2 cup brown rice rinsed
- 2 tsp olive oil
- 1-1/4 cups chicken broth, low-sodium
- 1/2 tsp turmeric powder
- 1/4 cup yellow onion, minced
- 1/2 tsp fresh garlic, minced
- salt

Instructions:

1. In a pot, heat the olive oil over medium-high heat.
2. Add the onion and garlic and cook until fragrant for about 3 minutes.
3. Pour the broth into a container when hot and add turmeric powder to it.
4. Add rice and chicken broth to a pot, cover, and lower the heat to low. Let simmer for 35 minutes or until done.
5. After 35 minutes, remove from heat but do not open the lid yet - let it sit with the lid on for an additional 10 minutes.
6. Fluff with a fork before serving and add salt to taste if desired.

Cauliflower Rice Substitute

Ingredients:

- 1 head of cauliflower (grate the cauliflower on the small grater holes to make a rice-type of consistency, making about 1 cup)
- 2 cups of fresh vegetable mix for stir-fry, chopped to about ½-inch pieces
- ¾ tsp garlic, chopped
- ½ tsp peeled ginger, grated
- 1 tsp low-sodium soy sauce
- 1/4 tsp Red pepper flakes

Instructions:

1. Heat a nonstick skillet to medium.
2. Add a bit of oil and put in the grated cauliflower and red pepper flakes.
3. Let it cook until the cauliflower is slightly browned.
4. This should take less than a minute.
5. Season with salt and set aside.
6. Using the same pan, add a little oil and stir-fry the mixed vegetables.
7. Cook until the vegetables are softened.
8. Move the vegetables to one side of the pan and sauté garlic and ginger until aromatic.

9. Add in the cooked cauliflower and stir everything including the vegetables.
10. Turn the heat off and add the tamari. Mix until everything is well-coated.
11. Season with salt to taste.
12. Add more pepper flakes if more spice is desired.

Conclusion

Congratulations on making it to the end of this guide! By now, you should have a good understanding of what the Rice Diet is and how it can help you manage chronic diseases such as hypertension, diabetes, and heart disease.

The Rice Diet's focus on whole, nutritious foods can help improve your overall health and well-being by reducing inflammation, promoting weight loss, and lowering your risk of developing chronic conditions.

Incorporating the Rice Diet into your lifestyle may take some effort and commitment, but the benefits are numerous. By making this dietary change, you can take control of your health and feel better. Managing chronic diseases requires a long-term approach, and the Rice Diet is a sustainable option that you can stick to for years to come.

It's important to remember that changing your diet alone may not be enough to manage your chronic conditions. You should work with your doctor and healthcare team to develop a comprehensive treatment plan that works for you. Incorporating regular exercise into your routine, managing stress levels, and taking any prescribed medication will also play important roles in managing your chronic conditions.

If you're ready to give the Rice Diet a try, start by incorporating more plant-based foods, whole grains, and lean proteins into your meals. Gradually reducing processed and high-fat foods from your diet will also help. You can also seek the guidance of a registered dietitian or nutritionist to help you create a personalized meal plan that meets your dietary needs and preferences.

Remember that making small, sustainable changes over time is the key to success. It's okay to slip up occasionally, but try to get back on track as soon as possible, and don't beat yourself up over it. With time and consistency, you'll see improvements in your health and well-being.

In conclusion, the Rice Diet is a promising solution for individuals who are looking to improve their health outcomes and manage chronic diseases. By focusing on whole, unprocessed foods and reducing inflammation in the body, the Rice Diet can help you achieve a healthier and happier life. With a little effort and commitment, you can take control of your health and start feeling better today.

FAQs

What is the Rice Diet, and how does it work?

The Rice Diet is a simple, plant-based eating plan focused on low-sodium, low-fat, and high-fiber foods like rice, fruits, vegetables, and whole grains. It is designed to promote weight loss, lower blood pressure, improve heart health, and manage chronic conditions by encouraging nutrient-rich, natural foods.

Can the Rice Diet help manage chronic diseases?

Yes, the Rice Diet can help manage chronic diseases such as hypertension, diabetes, and heart disease. Its emphasis on low sodium, minimal fat, and whole foods can reduce inflammation, regulate blood sugar levels, and support cardiovascular health.

Is the Rice Diet safe for everyone with a chronic condition?

While the Rice Diet is generally considered safe, individuals with certain medical conditions—like advanced kidney disease or those requiring a specific nutrient balance—should consult a healthcare provider before starting. A dietitian can help customize the plan to meet individual needs.

Are there any risks or side effects of following the Rice Diet?

The Rice Diet is restrictive and may lead to nutritional deficiencies if followed long-term without guidance. Fat and protein intake is low, which can lead to fatigue for some people. Always ensure you're meeting your nutritional needs with the help of a professional.

What changes might I expect to see if I follow the Rice Diet?

Many people experience weight loss, lower blood pressure, better cholesterol levels, and improved blood sugar control. However, results vary based on overall health and adherence to the plan.

Are there specific types of rice or foods I should include?

Brown rice, wild rice, or other whole-grain rice varieties are preferred as they're more nutrient-dense than white rice. Pairing rice with fruits, vegetables, and legumes ensures you get a variety of vitamins, minerals, and fiber.

How do I incorporate the Rice Diet into my daily routine?

Start by planning meals around rice, vegetables, and fruits. Limit processed foods, sugar, and salt. Preparing meals in advance and experimenting with herbs and spices for flavor can make the diet easier to maintain. Small, gradual changes are often more sustainable than an immediate overhaul.

References and Helpful Links

Walter Kempner, MD - founder of the Rice Diet - Dr. McDougall. (2024, July 1). Dr. McDougall.
https://www.drmcdougall.com/education/information-all/walter-kempner-md-founder-of-the-rice-diet/

About chronic disease | Center for Managing Chronic Disease. (n.d.).
http://cmcd.sph.umich.edu/about/about-chronic-disease/

Rice Diet - The Residential Clinic. (n.d.).
https://www.ricedietprogram.com/r_test_over/

Silver, N. (2023, June 7). Can eating rice affect my diabetes? Healthline.
https://www.healthline.com/health/diabetes/diabetes-rice

Richards, L. (2024, June 14). What is the rice diet and does it have benefits? https://www.medicalnewstoday.com/articles/rice-diet

Contratto, A. W., & Rogers, M. B. (1948). The use of the rice diet in the treatment of hypertension in nonhospitalized patients. New England Journal of Medicine, 239(15), 531–536.
https://doi.org/10.1056/nejm194810072391501

Biswas, C. (2024, November 6). The rice Diet – How it works, what to eat, and benefits. STYLECRAZE.
https://www.stylecraze.com/articles/rice-diet/

Singh, A. N. (2024, August 11). How to eat rice on a weight-loss diet. Healthshots. https://www.healthshots.com/how-to/ways-to-eat-rice-on-weight-loss-diet/

Braverman, J., & EyeEm/EyeEm/GettyImages, K. S. /. (2023, February 1). The rice diet: What it is and whether you should try it. Livestrong.com. https://www.livestrong.com/article/478797-the-rice-diet-plan-menu/

www.ingramcontent.com/pod-product-compliance
Lightning Source LLC
LaVergne TN
LVHW012029060526
838201LV00061B/4529